Sun-damaged Skin

Sun-damaged Skin

Ronald Marks

Department of Dermatology
University of Wales College of Medicine
Cardiff, UK

Produced and published by Martin Dunitz Limited
for *ORTHO Division of Cilag Ltd*

Martin Dunitz

First published in the United Kingdom in 1992 by
Martin Dunitz Ltd, 7–9 Pratt Street, London NW1 0AE

ISBN 1-85317-099-2

Typeset by TecSet
Printed and bound in Singapore

Contents

Foreword

In this thin volume Professor Marks has once again demonstrated his extraordinary skill for condensing subjects of serious medical importance into crisp, clear and concise language that nevertheless does not trivialize scientific truth. In a mere five chapters, all richly illustrated with dramatic clinical photographs and vivid histologic examples of photodamaged skin, Marks has made it possible for the intelligent layman to learn the essential facts about solar radiation and its harmful effects on human skin. Best of all, his penchant for the practical and useful is evident in the two chapters that reaffirm the key missions of medical science, namely prevention and treatment of disease (in this case, photoaging).

No one who follows Marks's rules of protection from pointless and excessive sun exposure need develop the wretched appearance of premature aging, that truly ruined portrait of wrinkles, blotches and a yellow, sallow, leathery or dry surface in which are sprinkled a variety of neoplastic growths, certain ones of which can cause mutilation and death. Marks's common sense shines throughout: he does not prescribe living in darkness, offering instead simple modifications in behavior, aided by the great protection afforded by modern sunscreens – the choices here are very great, with formulations to suit every conceivable earthly need.

This is a fast-reading, trenchant text which can be strongly recommended for school teachers, outdoor sportsmen, educators who set public health policies in areas where cloud coverage is rare, first-year medical students, traveler-vacationists and last, but not least, mothers!

Albert M. Kligman, MD, PhD
Professor of Dermatology
University of Pennsylvania

Acknowledgement

I am very grateful to the Medical Illustration Department at the University of Wales College of Medicine for their help with the many photographs in this book, and to my secretarial staff for their excellent help and dedication in preparing the manuscript, and to my long-suffering wife, Hilary, for not complaining while I took the time to put it together.

RM

1

Solar Radiation and Susceptibility

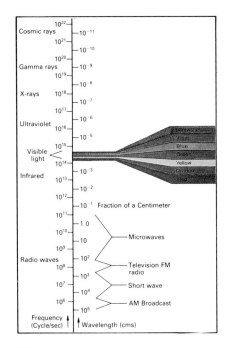

Figure 1.1

The solar spectrum. The visible portion can be seen to occupy just a small portion in the centre.

To many it may seem faintly ridiculous that exposure to the sun can be harmful. It seems natural to bask in its warmth and delight in the brightness and colour that it gives. Indeed, to some ancient peoples the sun became a god to thank for 'bountiful life', to sacrifice before to ensure good harvests, an object to love, fear and placate. It is certainly true that all life on the planet Earth stems from the energy in sunlight. Carbohydrates, rich in energy, are produced by plant photosynthesis; fossil fuels derive ultimately from plants that obtained their energy stores from sunshine. However, this same life-giving, friendly appearing object can also damage and destroy, and this book is essentially about its harmful effects on the skin.

Solar Irradiation

The sun emits a broad spectrum of electromagnetic energy (Fig. 1.1) which includes X-rays and radiowaves, but what mainly concerns us here is the segment of radiation which includes visible light, ultraviolet radiation (UVR) and infrared radiation

Figure 1.2

The visible and ultraviolet portions of the solar spectrum. The UV portion is normally divided into three segments: A is the long-wave portion; B is known as the erythemogenic portion; and C is the short-wave portion.

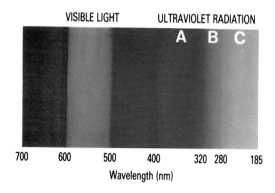

(Fig. 1.2). Because 'ultraviolet' is beyond violet, the longest wavelength for visible light, strictly speaking it is incorrect to speak of 'ultraviolet light' (although many persist in doing so!) and it is better to use the term 'radiation' to describe ultraviolet. The sun's spectrum is continuous in that all wavelengths are radiated, as opposed to some artificial sources of UVR which may give out their energy at particular wavelengths only.

The UVR part of the spectrum is conventionally and quite conveniently divided into three sections known as the short (UVC), medium (UVB) and long (UVA) parts of the UVR

spectrum. The wavelengths of these types of UVR are as follows: UVC, 200–280 nm; UVB, 280–315 nm; and UVA, 315–400 nm. The short-wave UVC section need concern us very little here as all of it is absorbed in the atmosphere—mainly by the ozone. Nonetheless, it should be noted that currently the ozone is under threat of destruction (see later) because of man-made gases finding their way into the atmosphere, and UVC could begin to have major biological importance for man. Sunburn is caused by UVB, and the medium waveband of UVR is sometimes called the 'erythematogenic' part of the spectrum because of

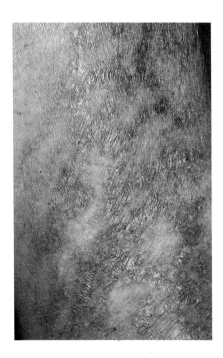

Figure 1.3

Reticulate pigmentation of the leg, due to erythema ab igne. This is caused by chronic heat injury from sitting in front of a focal source of heat such as a coal fire.

this. The bulk of chronic 'sun-damage', more correctly termed 'photodamage', is also caused by this part of the UVR spectrum. Long-wave UVR (UVA) is thought to have less

biological effect although wavelengths in this range are mainly responsible for various photosensitivities resulting from drugs or spontaneous disease. More importantly here, UVA is now recognized to have considerable importance as a cause of chronic photodamage to the skin.

The visible part of the solar spectrum seems quite benign to the skin although it is perhaps worthwhile remembering that the visible wavelengths can be made to damage the skin when manipulated in a laser system. In addition, visible light does appear to have sufficient energy to aggravate the uncommon and disabling skin condition known as actinic reticuloid.

Beyond the red portion of the visible light is the infrared part of the spectrum which has a strong heating effect and is above 700 nm. This is mentioned because infrared does seem to be a contributory factor in the production of chronic photodamage. Heating is known to be responsible for the disorder called erythema ab igne (Fig. 1.3) found on the lower legs of the elderly who warm themselves by sitting near a focal source of heat such as a coal or electric fire. Interestingly, biopsies of this condition show very similar tissue changes to those in chronic photodamage. The dermis shows a type of elastotic degenerative change (see page 14) and the epidermis may also demonstrate minor degrees of dysplasia quite like that observed in skin damaged by long-term exposure to the sun (Fig. 1.4).

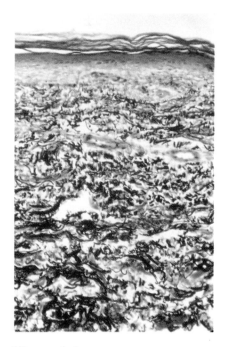

Figure 1.4

Histological section from erythema ab igne. In this photomicrograph the elastic staining material is seen in black thoughout the dermis.

Other Sources of Damaging Radiaton

Apart from the heating sources mentioned above there are other artificial sources that supply more damaging forms of energy. Probably the most important of these at the moment are the UVA suntan lamps found in salons in the high street and in sports complexes. Those apparatuses tan efficiently but they also damage the skin and it is odd that they are permitted to proliferate in the UK in an almost completely unregulated fashion. For example, it is estimated that in 1988 40 000 new salons opened and 80 000 domestic units were sold in the UK compared with 5000 units in 1982, and a recent survey found that 10% of the population of the UK and the Netherlands had visited a salon in the previous year, providing a substantial and unnecessary source of damage to the skin (15% of these were women between the ages of 16 and 30).

Skin diseases such as psoriasis, atopic dermatitis and mycosis fungoides are often treated by UVR in one form or another. Photochemotherapy with UVA (PUVA), in which the reaction of the skin is heightened by the use of a photosensitizing drug such as 8-methoxypsoralen, is the most frequently used form of UVR. These treatments are often successful and are quite popular. The potentially harmful effect of therapeutically administered UVR is well recognized and the use of UVR is justified only after due consideration of the risk–benefit ratio by the prescribing dermatologist and after discussion with the patient concerned.

Of course, only a very small proportion of the population is treated with PUVA or some other form of UVR, but we are all exposed to fluorescent lamps at work or in the home. These do give out a small amount of UVR but the potential damage sustained from these sources seems to be of a low order and of no practical importance.

Finally, in discussing artifical sources it ought to be said that it is possible to be quite severely damaged from UVR encountered in the workplace. Notably, arc welding involves potential exposure to a significant amount of UVR. Germicidal lamps, laboratory sources of UVR and UVR sources employed in production of plastics are other potential sources of danger.

Sites of Photodamage

Clearly, the sites of damage are those that are persistently exposed to the sun. However, there are some particular points that are worth making. For example, bald scalp skin provides an easy target for incident solar radiation and one that frequently sustains severe solar damage and provides unpleasant clinical problems. The tops of the ears and the lower lip are other sites that sustain quite severe solar damage out of proportion to the rest of the facial skin. The same is true for the skin of the back of the neck which is particularly exposed in men employed in the building industry, in sailors and fishermen and in those who work in agriculture. The lower legs receive a surprising amount of solar radiation—presumably because they are also readily irradiated by UVR reflected by the floor or surface on which the legs are standing. Trousers protect the skin of the legs and it is only women in skirts who are prone to develop solar-induced skin cancers on the lower legs.

Inherent Protection and Susceptibility to UVR Damage

The amount of damage sustained from solar injury depends on two major factors—the dose of UVR received and the inherent protection of the individual concerned. The inherent protection of an individual depends on two factors. The first of these is the degree of skin pigmentation.

Skin pigmentation

The skin pigment concerned is the complex quinone polymer called melanin which is synthesized in the melanocytes that reside in the basal layer of the epidermis (Fig. 1.5). The initial chemical 'building-block' is the amino acid tyrosine which is converted to dihydroxyphenylalanine (DOPA) and thence to DOPA quinone by the enzymes tyrosinase and DOPA oxidase, respectively. The melanin that is synthesized is deposited on cellular organelles known as

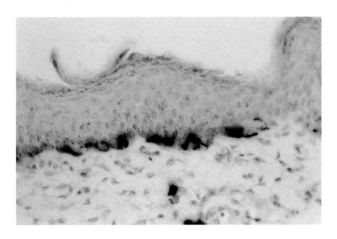

Figure 1.5

Section of normal skin prepared to show melanocytes in the basal layer, using the dihydroxyphenylalanine oxidase method. The black cells at the base of the epidermis show a positive reaction indicating that they are melanocytes.

melanosomes which aggregate as melanin particles. Melanin particles, once synthesized, are transferred from the melanocytes to surrounding keratinocytes via the dendritic processes of the pigment cells. Racial variations in pigment are due to variations not in the number of melanocytes present but in the activity of these cells. Melanin is brown–black although there are varieties that have a redder hue (phaeomelanin). The blackness of the melanin is due to its absorption of the visible light incident on it and its importance here is the fact that it absorbs UVR as well. The darker the skin, the greater its melanin content and the greater the resistance to solar injury.

The degree of protection provided by the melanin pigmentary system depends on the amount of melanin synthesized, on the size and shape of the melanosomes and on melanin particles and on their distribution in the keratinocytes. An individual's pigmentation is mostly determined genetically, but the degree of pigmentation can also be locally influenced. Factors that are injurious to the skin when applied at a low dose rate insufficient to produce acute and devastating damage tend to produce both epidermal thickening and an increased degree of melanin pigmentation. The stimuli that do this include persistent mechanical injury (rubbing and scratching), persistent low-grade heat injury (e.g. the condition of erythema ab igne, and injury from UVR (suntan)). A suntan will certainly help protect against further UVR damage but only to a

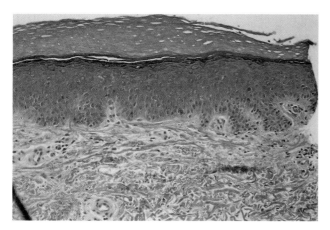

Figure 1.6

Section showing irregularly thickened epidermis with hyperkeratosis on the back of the exposed skin of the wrist in a 60-year-old man. The epidermis is on average some nine cells thick compared to three to five normally.

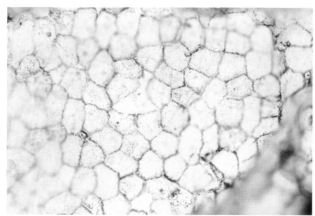

Figure 1.7

A strip of stratum corneum removed by the technique of skin surface biopsy using a cyanoacrylate adhesive, stained by the silver staining technique to show melanin pigment. This can be seen as small black dots within the individual cells.

degree dependent on the depth of pigmentation and the dose of UVR received. It is, for example, not impossible for a darkly pigmented black person to become sunburnt if a very high dose of UVR is allowed to reach the skin.

Stratum corneum and hair

When injured by UVR the epidermis proliferates and then thickens (Fig. 1.6). The epidermal thickening is accompanied by mild hyperkeratosis and this thickened stratum corneum

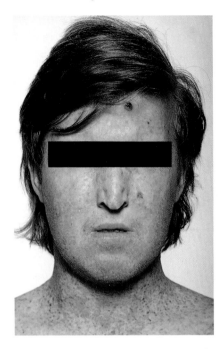

Figure 1.8

Young man with xeroderma pigmentosum. Notice the lesion on the forehead which turned out to be a squamous cell carcinoma. (Reproduced with kind permission from Dr Barry Statham.)

UVR. It has been computed that the normal stratum corneum is equivalent to a sunscreen with a protection factor (SPF) of 2 (see page 59). Hair also provides a degree of physical protection on the scalp and neck in most women. In men the degree of protection provided by the scalp hair is dependent on the presence of pattern alopecia as well as the vagaries of fashion.

Inherent UVR susceptibility

Although the degree of skin, eye and hair pigmentation is a fairly good guide to the way an individual reacts to the sun, susceptibility to UVR damage does not always parallel skin colour. The most dramatic example of this is the group of recessively inherited disorders known as xeroderma pigmentosum. In xeroderma pigmentosum there is an abnormality in the DNA repair mechanism. Normally when UVR damages nuclear DNA the damaged segments are excised enzymically after a few hours away from UVR and then replaced by new molecules. The process is actually quite complex and multistage, so that xeroderma pigmentosum in fact represents a series of similar recessively inherited abnormalities of DNA 'dark repair'. Affected individuals suffer severe sun damage and start to develop skin tumours of all types at a very early age, to which they often succumb (Fig. 1.8).

also supplies some protection against solar UVR. Of course, the horn cells (corneocytes) have melanin particles within them (Fig. 1.7) from the original donation to the keratinocytes from melanocytes at the base of the epidermis. However, even without melanin the horny layer absorbs some

Table 1.1 Genodermatoses in which there is abnormal light sensitivity.

Disorder	Comment
Xeroderma pigmentosum	A group of disorders in which there is an abnormality of repair to nuclear DNA after UVR damage
Rothmund–Thomson syndrome	Rare, recessive, multisystem disorder with characteristic facies and tendency to develop warty lesions at various sites which can become malignant
Bloom's syndrome	Unusual recessive disorder characterized by small stature and light-sensitive, telangiectatic skin. Increased chromosomal abnormalities and 'sister chromatid exchanges'. Metabolic fault unknown
Cockayne's syndrome	Very rare, recessive, multisystem disorder—may occur in association with xeroderma pigmentosum. May show premature aging. Metabolic basis unknown
Hartnup disease	A rare 'familial' pellagra-like syndrome characterized by erythema and other changes on sun-exposed skin, a cerebellar ataxia and a renal tubular reabsorptive defect of amino acids also present in the intestine
Porphyrias	A group of inherited disorders of synthesis of haem, resulting in accumulation of different porphyrins causing marked photosensitivity

There are other genodermatoses which have photosensitivity as part of their clinical picture (Table 1.1). Among these are rare conditions such as the Rothmund-Thomson syndrome, Bloom's syndrome and Cockayne's syndrome. The metabolic faults in these disorders have not been fully characterized but it is interesting to note that neoplastic lesions are more common in at least two of these genodermatoses.

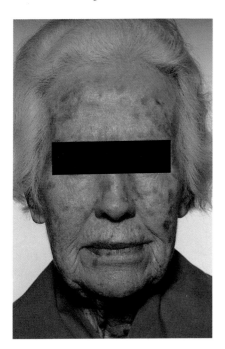

Figure 1.9

Severe solar damage. The numerous brown and pink patches are senile lentigines and solar keratoses, respectively (see later).

Apart from individuals with these specific and reasonably well character-ized disorders there are other groups whose sun sensitivity appears to be excessive and out of step with their skin, eye and hair colour. Topical application or ingestion of photosensi-tizing compounds (e.g. the psoralens) will certainly result in hypersensitivity to sunlight but there are others who are very sensitive to the sun and who have not been chemically photosensi-tized in any way. For example, Okla-homa Indians seem particularly prone to sun damage. The same is true of Celtic peoples no matter where they have ended up geographically. This group is well known to be prone to skin cancer in sunny and temperate cli-mates alike. They are recognized as being vulnerable in Australia, the southern USA and South Africa as well as in their native areas of Scot-land, Ireland and Wales. Part of this predisposition to solar damage is un-doubtedly related to the lack of pig-mentation of these individuals but it does not seem likely that this is the entire answer. Figures 1.9 and 1.10 show two patients of Welsh ancestry who have always lived in Cardiff, as housewives, have never had holidays abroad and who have never been 'sun worshippers'. They demonstrate marked solar damage out of propor-tion to their estimated cumulative UVR dose.

A recently completed survey of the population over the age of 60 in South Glamorgan, Wales revealed that solar keratoses (see page 37) occurred in approximately 20% of those seen. There seems to be a similarly high prevalence of premalignant lesions as well as non-melanoma skin cancer in Scotland and Ireland. Indeed, a group in Glasgow investigated the possibility of there being a predisposing metabo-lic abnormality that was responsible for the large numbers of solar ker-atoses in their patients. Their studies

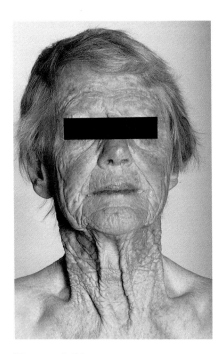

Figure 1.10

Severe photodamage affecting the face and neck. The skin of the latter is discoloured and sagging due to solar elastotic degenerative change.

showed a similar abnormality in DNA repair to that recognized in xeroderma pigmentosum but much less marked.

Skin type

In recent years it has become customary to divide people into groups according to the way they react to the sun. The system was devised by Dr T Fitzpatrick and his colleagues from Boston and so is known as the Boston skin-type classification. It is based on answers to the direct questions, 'Do you burn in the sun?' and 'Do you tan after being in the sun?'. The different groups and the criteria involved are set out in Table 1.2. Type I subjects—those who always burn and never tan—are mostly fair-skinned and have blonde hair with either blue or grey eyes. There is more variability about the depth of pigmentation of Types II and III, although Type II subjects tend to be fairer with chestnut and light-brown hair, and Type III are

Table 1.2 Skin types.

Skin type	Response to the questions 'Do you burn in the sun?' 'Do you tan after being in the sun?'
I	Always burn, never tan
II	Sometimes burn, never tan
III	Never burn, sometimes tan
IV	Never burn, always tan
V	Asian subjects
VI	Black African subjects

mostly subjects with darker-brown hair. Type IV subjects, those who never burn and always tan, mostly have dark-brown or black hair.

This skin typing is generally useful in indicating an individual's sun sensitivity but is by no means infallible as it relies on subjective responses. It seems to be more reliable than skin and hair colour for predictive purposes as far as sunburn is concerned, but we can only guess at how reliable it is with regard to chronic photodamage and skin cancer. More recently it has been suggested that a better way of categorizing susceptibility is actually to submit the individual to test doses of UVR on small areas of skin.

Social Trends

It has been suggested that in the past two or three decades the average UK citizen has received two to three times more UVR per annum than was previously the case. The seeds of the change were probably even earlier. Developing a suntan suddenly seemed to be 'the thing to do' in the 1920s when the smart young (and rich) set desported themselves on the beaches and yachts of the South of France. The golden-brown look indicated a fashionable, desirable and chic lifestyle and, like the Charleston, may have been a welcome reaction to the stuffiness that abounded in the early years of the twentieth century. However desirable, getting a tan was an expensive thing to do. It meant not working for a week or two and going somewhere sunny. It was not until the 1960s that getting a suntan was in reach of an appreciable segment of the population in northwest Europe. Increasing affluence with higher salaries and more time off work compounded with cheaper air travel to encourage the growth of the Mediterranean holiday resort. Two weeks 'soaking up the sun' became *de rigueur* and despite current economic ills the trend to spending more time in the sun seems to continue. Greater leisure time has also been accompanied by an increasing realization of the overall benefit from outdoor exercise. Inevitably this has been accompanied by further exposure of the skin to solar UVR. Whilst from most points of view these changes must be counted as beneficial to human development, they have overall been harmful to the skin!

2

Aging and Photodamage

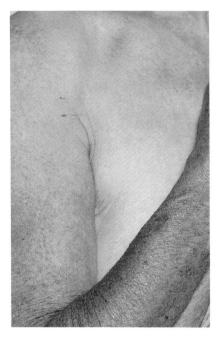

All living things age. The purpose and the mechanisms of this aging process are less well understood than the clinical phenomena that accompany it. Currently there are major research efforts underway trying to determine whether there is an inbuilt obsolescence programme within the complex instructions of DNA or whether molecules generated during metabolism or clones of abnormal lymphocytes irreversibly damage the complex cellular machinery. Aging of this inevitable sort is sometimes known as intrinsic aging to distinguish it from alterations that occur with the passage of time and are due to damage from external agencies, known as extrinsic aging. This distinction is not academic as far as skin is concerned, as can be seen in

Figure 2.1(a)

Photodamaged skin seen against non-exposed upper chest in late middle-aged woman. The exposed skin is hyperpigmented and thickened while the non-exposed skin is clearly different and paler.

Figs 2.1 (a) and (b). The sun-exposed areas of skin show changes that we associate with aging but are actually due to cumulated damage from the sun and other climatic stimuli. These changes in the skin have come to be known, somewhat inaccurately, as photoaging.

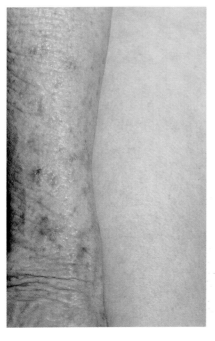

Figure 2.1(b)

Photodamaged skin of forearm seen against upper thigh and flank in 70-year-old female patient. The back of the forearm shows the changes of severe photodamage with some dyspigmentation, wrinkling and purpuric lesions.

As they are not, as far as we know, anything to do with the biological process of aging they are better described as 'photodamage'. The relevance, of course, is that we can certainly do something about preventing photodamage and may even be able to ameliorate photodamage once it has already developed.

Aging is not a popular phenomenon. For the most part the elderly citizen is strikingly disadvantaged and the older he or she looks, the greater the problem. It need hardly be said that this is the basis of a vast industry ranging from cosmetic surgery at one end of the spectrum to quack rejuvenation claims at the other. Somewhere along the line joining these two extremes there are all the cosmetic manoeuvres adopted by women (and increasingly men) to appear younger, including hair dyeing, colour cosmetics and emollients. The fact that so much money is spent on trying to look younger indicates the general importance of not appearing aged.

Dermal Alterations in Photodamage

The major cause of the changed appearance due to photodamage is the alteration in the dermal connective tissue known as solar elastotic degenerative change. This is an odd response of the dermal fibroblast to the damaging influence of UVR in which an abnormal dermal connective tissue is synthesized which has the staining qualities of elastic tissue (Fig. 2.2). How this occurs is uncertain, as most of the damaging UVR does not reach down in the dermis where the bulk of the change is found. It has been

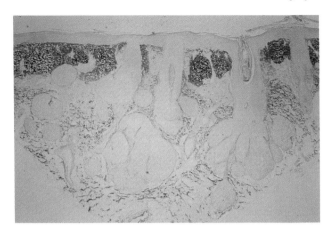

Figure 2.2

Histological section prepared to demonstrate elastotic degenerative change using an elastic tissue stain (orcein stain). The dark areas subepidermally represent elastic tissue.

suggested that the alteration to the synthetic profile of the dermal fibroblast is the result of damage to the epidermis, with release of cytokines from the keratinocytes that diffuse down and secondarily influence the cells of the dermis. Longer-wave UVR penetrates deeper into the skin and some of the damage may well be due to the direct effects of UVA on the cells of the dermis. The truth is that we are not certain which part of the solar UVR spectrum is responsible for which and how much of the changes observed in photodamaged skin—and as pointed out in the last chapter (see page 3), focal heating sources certainly cause elastotic degenerative change and it may well be that solar infrared also contributes to the production of the abnormal elastotic tissue.

In routine histological tissues stained with haematoxylin and eosin, the abnormal elastotic tissue tends to be more basophilic than normal and loses the normal fibrillar structure of dermal connective tissue to take on either a characteristic 'chopped spaghetti' appearance or a homogeneous, almost cartilaginous appearance (Fig. 2.3). Occasionally areas of inflammation and foci of macrophages and giant cells are found in the presence of severe solar elastosis. The cause of these actinic granulomas is unknown and they do not appear to be associated with any clinical sequelae. The abnormal dermal connective tissue also becomes patchily coated with IgG, and once again the significance of this is uncertain.

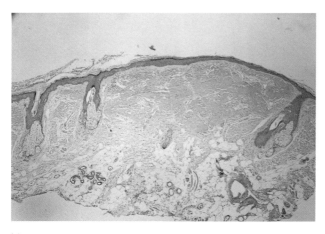

(a)

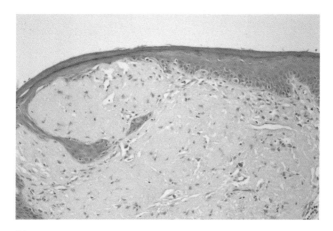

(b)

Figure 2.3

(a) Section demonstrating considerable elastotic degenerative change in the upper mid dermis. The affected tissue is basophilic and disorganized. (b) Elastotic degenerative change in the upper and mid dermis. The affected tissue is basophilic but homogeneous in appearance, rather than disorganized and 'chopped spaghetti-like' as in (a). Note also that there are some inflammatory cells scattered within the abnormal tissue.

Clinical Signs due to Solar Elastosis

Not everyone who has solar elastotic degenerative change has the same clinical sequelae (Table 2.1) and why this is the case is not clear. A frequently observed change is one that the author terms the 'sallow' appearance (Fig. 2.4). Patients who show this change have a uniform, pale sallow lemon-yellow tint to their skin, the exact cause of which is uncertain. Another variety of clinical appearance due to solar damage is the 'English rose complexion'. Although the pop-

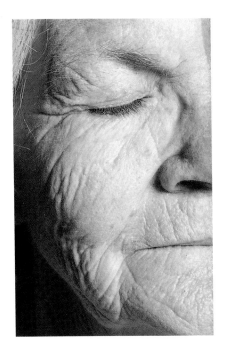

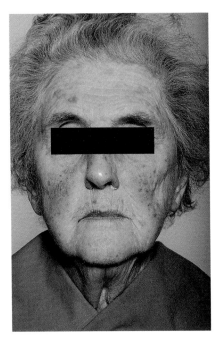

Figure 2.4

Severe photodamage in an elderly patient. The affected skin demonstrates a sallow, dusky yellow–brown appearance. This patient also shows extensive wrinkling.

Figure 2.5

Patient with features of moderately severe photodamage, showing pink cheeks with telangiectasia due to the underlying vasodilatation permitted by the elastotic degenerative change.

ular view is that pink cheeks denote health, they may indicate only that their owner has sustained a significant degree of solar damage (Fig. 2.5). An extension of this mild abnormality is what is sometimes known as 'farmer's face' in which there is marked telangiectasia all over the cheeks (Fig. 2.6). These physical signs of erythema and telangiectasia probably result from the lack of support for the dermal vasculature from the surrounding dermal connective tissue (Fig. 2.7) but why they occur in some but not all sun-damaged individuals is mysterious.

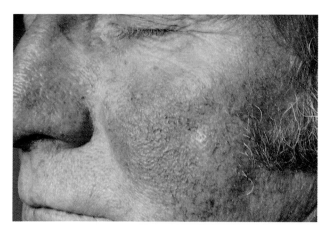

Figure 2.6

Erythema and telangiectasia in a farm worker due to severe elastotic degenerative change.

Table 2.1 Physical signs of solar elastotic degenerative change.

Sign	Explanation
Sallow dusky yellowish discolouration of skin	Altered optical properties of skin
Telangiectasia and redness of cheeks	Persistent vasodilatation of subpapillary venous plexus resulting from deficient perivascular connective tissue support
Senile purpura	Minor trauma to vulnerable dilated vessels and deficient macrophage function
Fine lines and wrinkles	Altered mechanical properties of dermis
Triradiate (stellate) scars	Probably precipitated by minor trauma but exact cause unknown

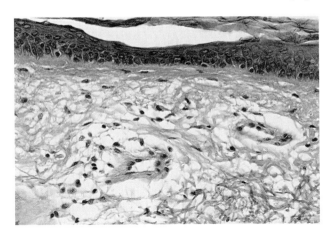

Figure 2.7

Histological section showing severe elastotic degenerative change with telangiectasia and lack of perivascular supportive connective tissue.

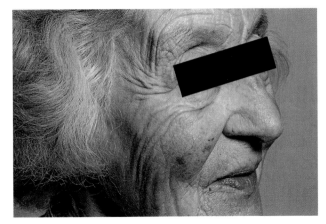

Figure 2.8

Facial wrinkles due to solar elastotic change. Note the severe changes around the eyes.

The abnormal dermal connective tissue does not have the same mechanical qualities that normal connective tissue has, and this probably accounts for the various creases and lines observed on the photodamaged face. Not all lines and furrows are due to photodamage. Some are due to habit, such as the furrows on the forehead—it would be interesting to contrast the number of these in senior medical academics with the numbers in other groups of physicians! Others seem to be in part the result of inherent tissue laxity and in part the result of gravity—those in the

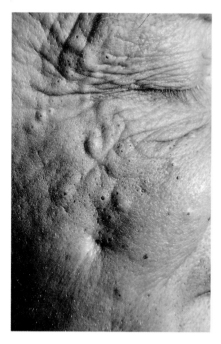

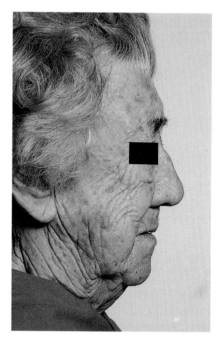

Figure 2.9

Very severe solar elastotic change around the upper part of the face, especially at the external angle of the eye – known colloquially as 'crow's feet'.

Figure 2.10

Extensive lines and wrinkles on the face of an elderly lady due to photodamage.

nasolabial grooves are probably of this kind and seem comparable to the jowls of the bloodhound.

Crease lines or wrinkles from photodamage are first observed around the eyes (Fig. 2.8). They are seen in particular beneath the eyes, on the lower eyelids. However, they are most noticeable at the sides of the eyes, particularly when the individual smiles and 'wrinkles up' the upper facial muscles (Fig. 2.9). These marks radiating from the external angle of the eye are the dreaded and appropriately named 'crow's feet' so feared by women approaching middle-age.

A visitor from space would not have imagined that such a minor physical change could cause so much distress and apparent disability. Clearly it

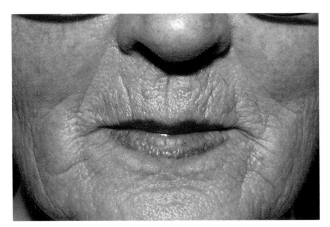

Figure 2.11

Severe photodamage of the lower face showing lines radiating from the lips. This pattern of change has been thought to be partly due to smoking but this has not been confirmed.

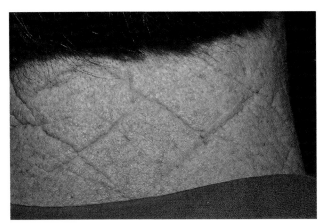

Figure 2.12

Severe elastotic change on the back of the neck in a manual labourer. This condition is known as cutis rhomboidalis nuchae, or colloquially as 'sailor's neck'.

does, and it is not difficult to find a reasonable explanation. As mentioned above, society does not value or respect the aged look and this tendency with its sexual overtones is heightened by an advertising industry that promotes a smooth youthful look as being the only attractive image worth pursuing.

As the degree of photodamage increases, the number of lines on facial skin increases, until in the worst cases the entire face is covered by numerous short wrinkles (Figs 2.10 and 2.11).

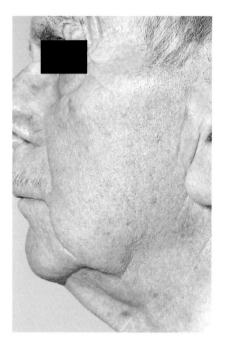

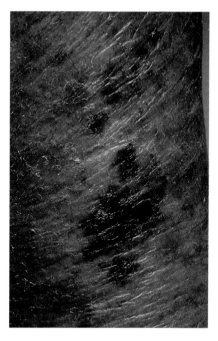

Figure 2.13

Laxity of the skin of the neck due at least in part to solar elastotic change.

Figure 2.14

So-called senile purpura on the back of the forearm of an elderly man. This is invariably associated with solar elastosis.

On the back of the neck these fine wrinkles are not found; instead, a deeper system of furrows develops. These furrows are often arranged in a rhomboidal pattern (Fig. 2.12) and because the affected skin often has a reddish hue the individuals who have developed this condition have come to be known as 'red-necks'. As the condition is common and severe in agricultural and building-site la-bourers whose necks are easily damaged by the sun as they work, the term 'red-neck' has become pejorative and derisive. Another frequently used term for the condition is 'sailor's neck', which seems less likely to offend than the one above and cer-tainly easier to remember than the Latin tag, cutis rhomboidalis nuchae. The scalp does not seem to wrinkle, and this is presumably because of its

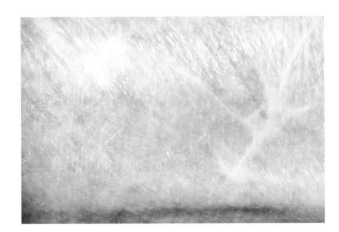

Figure 2.15

Stellate scar (tri-radiate scar) on the back of the forearm in an individual with severe elastotic degenerative change.

taut bound-down nature. Skin on the neck does wrinkle but often hangs down in folds in the elderly due to laxness, especially in the obese, so that the small wrinkle lines are overshadowed by the dewlaps (Fig. 2.13).

Quite large persistent bruises are often seen in photodamaged subjects on the backs of the hands and the exposed parts of the extensor aspects of the forearms (Fig. 2.14). These patches of so-called senile purpura seem to be due to the lack of protective connective tissue around the vulnerable vessels so that they are easily injured after relatively minor trauma. They remain for long periods because of the depressed function of elderly macrophages. In addition to these changes, solar elastosis is also strongly associated with an odd type of scar known as the stellate scar. These

curious angulated lesions are found mainly on the back of the forearm (Fig. 2.15). They seem to be produced by relatively trivial trauma and their unusual and distinctive clinical appearance is difficult to explain.

It is often said that sun-damaged skin has a leathery look and feel: it is certainly thicker than normal, non-sun-damaged skin. Its physical properties differ too, accounting for the different texture and the different behaviour of skin with solar elastosis when it is stretched or pinched. Both the elastic properties and the viscous properties are changed and the breaking strength is less. These clinical and physical alterations are due to the reduction in collagen and the increase in elastin and proteoglycan in the abnormal tissue.

The Photodamaged Epidermis

The epidermis is made up mainly of keratinocytes (Fig. 2.16) but also has melanin-producing melanocytes in the basal layer and the Langerhans' cells, which trap, process and present antigen, scattered in the malpighian layer. All these cell types show signs of photodamage. In covered parts the epidermis gradually thins during intrinsic aging but in exposed areas of skin the epidermis is variably thickened (Fig. 2.17). The rate of cell production is also increased in the exposed skin compared to similar non-exposed sites. The stratum corneum may also be a little thicker in chronically sun-exposed sites.

The melanocytes are also increased in sun-exposed skin but in badly photodamaged areas they are patchily increased, accounting for the pigment blotchiness sometimes seen in photodamaged skin. Langerhans' cells do not share in the hyperplastic response of the epidermis. They seem to reduce in numbers, although elegant experiments in patients receiving PUVA treatment suggest that Langerhans' cell function is affected more than the proportion of these cells in the epidermis. The reduction in number (or function) has important implications. It is accompanied by a reduction in cellular immunocompetence. It is, for example, more difficult to be sensitized to a test potent sensitizer on skin that has been experimentally irradiated. As this type of depressed delayed hypersensitivity is accompanied by an increased chance of developing skin cancer, the diminution in Langerhans' cell function may be one mechanism of UV carcinogenesis.

Apart from epidermal hyperplasia the epidermis shows one other important alteration. This is epidermal dysplasia, and is the forerunner of neoplastic change. The first changes to be noticed are minor irregularities in cell and nuclear size, shape and staining. The cells also seem to lose the strict vertical orientation associated with normal differentiation, and a loss of polarity results (Fig. 2.18). Occasionally epidermal thinning occurs against a background of hyperplasia elsewhere.

This minimal dysplastic change is present in clinically normal (but sun-damaged) skin. In its minor degrees it requires some practice to recognize but when severe it is not difficult to identify. One stage further down the line histologically is the solar keratosis—it is uncertain whether in fact there is a continuum from the minimal dysplastic change condition to solar keratosis or whether a separate 'event' must take place before the premalignant keratosis arises.

Do the hyperplastic and minimal dysplastic states of the epidermis cause any clinical change? Probably they result in subtle pigmentary and textural alterations but these have not been adequately characterized. Surface markings are decreased and more irregular on markedly photodamaged

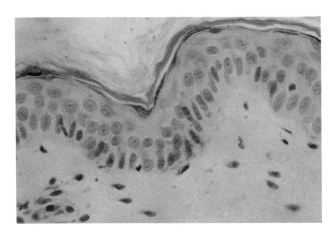

Figure 2.16

Histological section of normal epidermis, which is on average three to five cells thick.

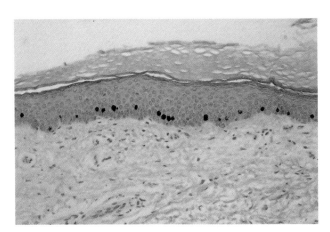

Figure 2.17

Section showing irregularly thickened epidermis on the back of the forearm of an elderly female patient. The blackened cells at the base of the epidermis have been labelled by the process of autoradiographic labelling with [^{3}H]thymidine and are present in increased numbers.

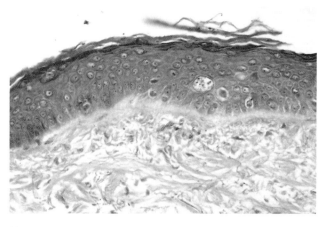

(a)

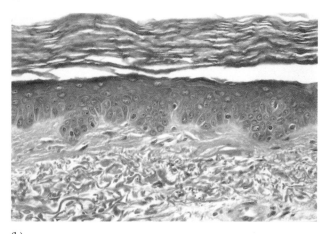

(b)

Figure 2.18

(a) Histological section from photo-damaged site on the back of the forearm showing some cellular irregularity and loss of cell polarity as signs of minimal epidermal dysplasia. (b) Section showing considerable irregularity in epidermal profile and some loss of cell polarity, characteristic of minimal epidermal dysplasia.

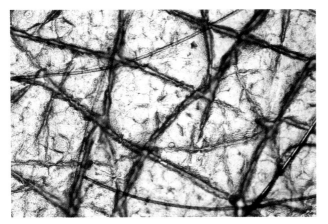

(a)

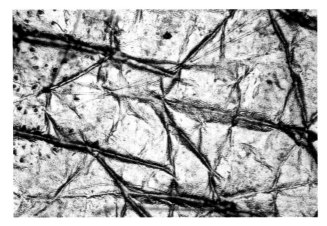

(b)

Figure 2.19

(a) Stratum corneum from the back of the right hand of a man of 39, showing the normal rhomboidal pattern. (b) Stratum corneum from the back of the hand of a man of 75 who was considerably photodamaged. There is some loss of skin surface markings and irregularity in pattern typical of chronic photodamage.

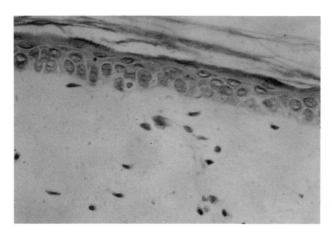

Figure 2.20

Histological section showing marked epidermal atrophy in a non-exposed site from the arm of a woman of 85. The epidermis is on average two cells thick and the epidermal cells are smaller than normal.

skin (Fig. 2.19). The reason for this is not clear, but presumably it has to do with the altered epidermal structure and function.

Intrinsic Aging

Because of the popularity of sun-bathing and 'healthy' outdoor sports in recent years it is difficult to be certain that any area of skin is completely undamaged by previous sun exposure. Buttock skin is probably the least damaged but in recent years even this once very private area somehow gets suntanned. Nonetheless, some alterations seem to be due primarily to the aging process itself rather than to any identifiable external agency. All parts of the skin seem to experience changes due to the intrinsic process but only some of these can be described here.

Epidermal changes

The epidermis gradually thins due to a decrease in the number of epidermal cells in its thickness, as well as a decrease in epidermal cell size (Fig. 2.20). Interestingly, the stratum corneum does not share in this process of attrition, and is not distinguishable as being elderly when histological sections are examined microscopically (Fig. 2.21). Stratum corneum does not change markedly in its barrier function with increasing age—perhaps an indication of the importance of this property to any form of independent existence. Indeed, some barrier functions, such as that against trans-epidermal water loss, seem to be more efficient in elderly skin (see below). There are, however, alterations in the horny layer both in structure and function. Structurally there is a diminution in the fine surface markings

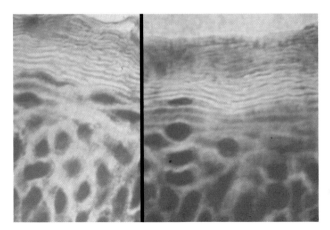

Figure 2.21

Composite photomicrograph of skin to show the structure of the stratum corneum in a non-exposed site from the upper arm of a man of 95 (*left*) and a similar site in a man of 21 (*right*). There is no major difference.

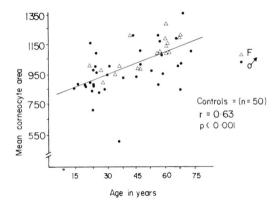

Figure 2.22

Mean corneocyte area plotted against age of 50 normal subjects from non-exposed sites on the flexor aspect of the forearm, showing linear relationship between age and mean corneocyte area.

although not to the same extent as in photodamaged skin. Several groups of investigators have noted that the mean surface area of corneocytes is linearly correlated with age—the older the individual, the greater the mean surface area of his or her corneocytes (Fig. 2.22). The thickness of corneocytes is much less easy to measure but

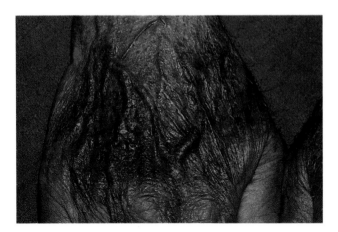

Figure 2.23
Marked skin thinning in an elderly man. Note the prominence of the veins in this elderly subject due to the greatly thinned skin.

what few observations there are on corneocyte volume suggest that this parameter also increases with age. The increased area indicates that there is a decrease in intercellular space per unit volume of stratum corneum and this may explain the decreased rate of transepidermal water loss in the elderly.

Desquamation also seems to be slowed in the elderly, though curiously this may not always be tied to changes in the rate of epidermal cell production. There are also alterations in the mechanical qualities of the stratum corneum of aging skin so that it becomes stiffer and less extensible and fractures at lower loads than in youth. It contains less water than young stratum corneum and this may account partly for its altered mechanical properties.

Dermal aging

Collagen becomes more insoluble and more extensively cross-linked with increasing age. There is also a gradual loss of interfibrillary proteoglycan. The net result of these and other changes is that the dermis becomes gradually thinner in the elderly—the rate of change being more marked in men (Fig. 2.23)—and the skin behaves differently when stretched. Skin is stiffer and less extensible in the elderly and deformations take much longer to regain normality. Pinching up a fold of skin, for example, gives some confirmation of this as the fold takes much longer to flatten in older individuals, although of course the subcutaneous tissue is also being tested here. Routine observation suggests that hair distribution, hair growth, sweat gland function, pigmentation and the response to wounding also all diminish in aging but further description is inappropriate here.

Assessment of Photodamage

Measurement of the degree of photodamage is useful for both individual patient management and as an essential part of a study of an agent designed to prevent or reverse photodamage. No single measurement technique can provide all the data necessary. In the first place, individual susceptibility dictates that the physical signs of photodamage differ in extent and severity. Some subjects become very wrinkled, for example, whilst others do not but develop marked telangiectasia even though they have had similar sun exposure. Furthermore, individual assessment techniques are for the most part insufficiently sensitive or reproducible to make just one sort of evaluation adequate. Amongst the most useful of the assessment methods available are techniques based on skin surface contour measurement. Image analysis of replicas taken in a standardized manner from the area of skin just lateral to the eye allows evaluation of the 'crow's foot' wrinkling at this site. Simpler but more time-consuming and more difficult to interpret are assessments of wrinkling using mechanical profilometers.

There are now several devices available that are capable of assessing the mechanical properties of skin *in vivo*. They measure the resistance of the skin to linear extension, to twisting or to elevation, depending on their design. Obtaining useful data from these techniques depends on a rigorous protocol to ensure complete standardization, and some knowledge of the significance of the measurements made. Ultrasound, using high-output transducers of frequencies in the region of 15 MHz and either the pulsed A-scan mode or the B-scan imaging mode, is not only able to measure the thickness of skin but can also determine the extent of solar elastosis.

The above non-invasive techniques cannot at the moment give useful information on the presence of changes in the epidermis and if this is required then skin biopsy and histological study are needed. Very small amounts of tissue are required and 3 or 4 mm diameter trephine biopsies are adequate and acceptable to most patients. The difficulty comes in quantifying the changes of interest. Epidermal thickness is relatively easy to assess since it needs only simple projection or image analysis techniques. Epidermal dysplasia has proved very difficult to quantify and at present the best approach is the use of visual analogue scales by trained observers under standardized conditions.

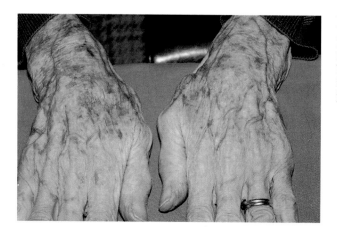

Figure 2.24

Numerous senile lentigines on the backs of the hands in an elderly subject.

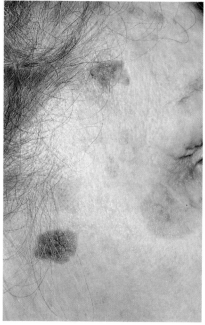

(a)

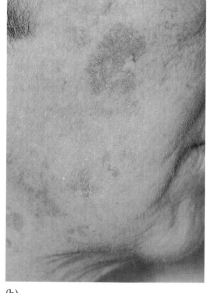

(b)

Figure 2.25

(a) A middle-aged woman with several brown patches on the right temple. Some of these are senile lentigines, others are seborrhoeic warts.

(b) Reddish-brown patch on the right cheek of a 60-year-old woman. It was difficult to say clinically whether this was a senile lentigine or a solar keratosis.

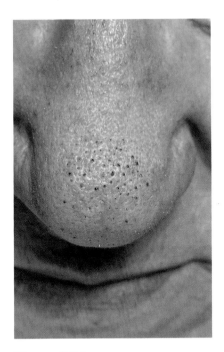 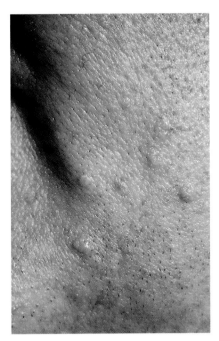

Figure 2.26

Senile comedones on the nose.

Figure 2.27

Dome-shaped pink papules of senile sebaceous gland hyperplasia. These lesions are sometimes mistaken for basal cell carcinoma.

Skin signs that may be due to photodamage

It seems fairly certain that ordinary seborrhoeic warts are not due to chronic photodamage but the same may not be true of the flat brown patches seen on the backs of the hands and the temples of the elderly (Fig. 2.24). These are sometimes called senile lentigines but the French have a better term for them, 'les medallions de cimitière' (cemetary medals). Recent histological studies suggest that these lesions, although similar clinically, may in fact be areas of epidermal dysplasia, true lentigines, flat seborrhoeic warts or even mixtures of these lesions (Fig. 2.25). They are certainly seen much more often on exposed areas of skin and are more common in sun-damaged subjects.

Senile comedones are other lesions that are found in areas of solar damage and have been thought to be due to photodamage (Fig. 2.26). Senile comedones also occur over the back and although it is true that these lesions are found on the upper cheeks in association with intense solar elastosis as part of a disorder described by Favre and Racouchot, one study did not find any striking association with solar elastosis. The same is true of sebaceous gland hyperplasia (Fig. 2.27) and it seems most unlikely that this disorder is associated with solar damage.

3

Skin Cancer

There can be no doubt that solar UVR is a potent carcinogenic agent. Skin cancer of all kinds is much more frequent in fair-skinned inhabitants of sunny countries such as Australia, South Africa and the southern USA and is seen predominantly on the light-exposed areas of skin. Furthermore, the greater the period and the intensity of exposure the greater the incidence of skin cancer. If any confirmation is necessary this is forthcoming from several sources. Firstly, there is abundant experimental evidence of the carcinogenic effect of UVR in animals. Then there is the unfortunate and inadvertent 'experiment' of PUVA in which patients with psoriasis were treated with long-wave (UVA) UVR and psoralens as photosensitizing agents to enhance the effect. Such patients have been found in some studies to develop skin cancers some 12 times more frequently than comparable control groups. Finally, patients with a disorder in which the usual capacity for nuclear DNA to repair itself after UVR damage is congenitally missing, known as xero-derma pigmentosum, are subject to the development of large numbers of skin cancers.

The relationship between UVR exposure and the development of squamous cell epithelioma is very good. It is not as good for basal cell carcinoma and malignant melanoma—both these lesions often occur on the covered parts—and clearly other aetiological agencies may be at work. Having said that, however, it has to be stated clearly that there has been a striking and steady increase in the numbers of patients with melanoma since records began in all communities whose inhabitants are predominantly fair-skinned Caucasians. In fact, there has been an approximate doubling of the numbers of patients each decade. Another quoted statistic is that there is a 6% increase per annum. The increase does seem to parallel the increase in affluence and leisure time of the Western World with its concomitant rush into the sun.

If the association between the increase in melanoma and the increased exposure to UVR is causal, what is the explanation for the fact that at least one-half of melanomas occur on parts of the skin not exposed to the sun? There have been several ingenious explanations for this inconvenient fact. The most convincing of these implicates the immunosuppression sustained from sun exposure but it also seems possible that melanocyte-stimulating and growth-promoting factors are liberated from exposed skin to act on melanocytes in covered sites.

One other finding is important: individuals who have been severely sunburnt on one or two occasions seem more prone to develop melanoma, suggesting that dose rate as well as total dose of UVR may be important.

Unfortunately, data for basal cell carcinoma are nowhere near as good as they are for melanoma: because of their frequency and non-lethal nature these carcinomas are rarely reported to cancer registries. They are extremely common—for example, they make up approximately 4% of all new patients with skin disorders seen at the University Hospital of Wales, Cardiff. The limited long-term sequential data that do exist suggest that there has been a steadily increasing number of patients with basal cell carcinoma over the past 25 years.

There have been interesting studies of the prevalence of premalignant epidermal lesions—solar keratoses and Bowen's disease. An Australian study of one community in sunny Queensland by Dr Robin Marks (colleague and friend, but not a relative) found a prevalence rate for solar keratoses in the population over the age of 40 of 54%. A survey of the population over the age of 60 in South Glamorgan found a corrected rate for solar keratoses of approximately 18%—unexpectedly high when the Welsh climate is considered! Although solar keratoses are often described as premalignant the rate of transformation of individual lesions is actually very low. Their main importance apart from their clinical inconvenience is that they indicate that the skin on which they arise has been significantly photodamaged and is capable of spawning frankly neoplastic lesions.

The details of the way in which solar UVR actually causes skin cancer have not been entirely worked out but several points are worth noting. In the first place solar UVR is thought to be a complete carcinogen as it both causes the initial damage and also promotes the formation of neoplastic lesions from the initiated sites, i.e. it is both an initiator and a promoter. This has some practical importance as it implies that protection from further UVR damage will reduce the chance of cancers arising from previously damaged skin. It is interesting to note that increases in the incidence of melanoma and solar keratoses have been noted just following periods of intense sunspot activity.

As to the actual details of the molecular events that underly photocarcinogenesis it is clear that several mechanisms are at work. In the first place it is known that pyrimidine dimers are formed from the DNA chains and that unless these are adequately corrected by the natural repair process errors in transcription will occur. It is also known that proto-oncogene activation occurs after UVR exposure and that as with some other neoplastic tissues there is accentuation of glucose-6-phosphate dehydrogenase metabolism.

From the above it will be clear that skin cancer is often the result of injudicious chronic solar exposure, that these disorders are quite common, and that their frequency is showing a frightening rate of increase. The question could well be asked, will the number of patients with skin cancer continue to grow? The gloomy answer is that it will, based on current trends and projections concerning alterations taking place in the environment.

There is no doubt that the ozone in the atmosphere is gradually being destroyed by chemical interaction with man-made gases that are either by-products of industry or specifically produced. The most notorious of the latter are the chlorofluorohydrocarbons used as aerosols, in refrigerators, for insulation and in air-conditioning units among other things. It has been estimated by the US Environmental Protection Agency that for each 1% depletion of the ozone layer one could expect an increase in the numbers of individuals who develop melanoma of 1–2%. The 'worst-case scenario' predictions for the year 2050 are horrifying. It is suggested that if there is no concerted global response to the warnings given, there could be a 50% depletion in the amount of ozone by the middle of the next century and that this would result in 18 000 extra melanomas and 12 million extra non-melanoma skin cancer cases in the existing population in the US.

Precursor Lesions of Non-melanoma Skin Cancer

As pointed out previously, chronically photodamaged skin often shows microscopic features of disordered epidermal growth and differentiation. This may not result in much in the way of clinical sequelae but suggests that the epidermis has started a journey along the path to neoplasia. Further along this path, visible 'preneoplastic' lesions occur known as solar keratoses. These are mostly small warty nodules or plaques (Figs 3.1 and 3.2) but also take the form of cutaneous horns (Fig. 3.3), scaling pink areas resembling discoid lupus erythematosus and known as lupoid or LE-like keratoses (Fig. 3.4) and pigmented lentigo-like lesions. As might be expected they are seen predominantly in areas of maximum photodamage such as the forehead, the bald scalp and the tops of the ears in men and the V of the neck and lower legs in women. Needless to say the clinical diagnosis is not always correct, and our experience and that of others suggest that the accuracy of diagnosis for this type of lesion is not better than 65%. The differential diagnosis includes seborrhoeic warts and viral warts (Table 3.1).

Histologically there is irregular epidermal thickening and loss of the usual regular epidermal differentiation, with parakeratosis and heterogeneity of cell and nuclear size, shape and staining reaction (Fig. 3.5). In many

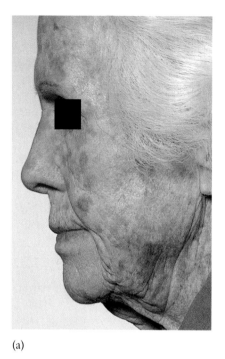

(a)

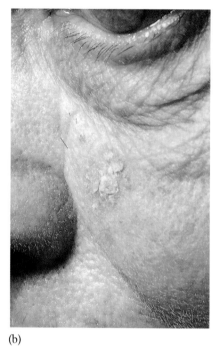

(b)

Figure 3.1

(a) Clusters of solar keratoses on the
cheek of an elderly woman.
(b) Solar keratosis on the cheek in
an elderly man.

Table 3.1 Differential diagnosis of warty lesion on the face or back or hands.

Diagnosis	Characteristic features
Solar (senile) keratosis	Localized pink scaling or hyperkeratotic papules or plaques
Seborrhoeic warts (basal cell papilloma)	Warty plaques tend to be pigmented, wartier and larger than solar keratoses
Viral warts	Tend to be more horny, less confined to sun-exposed sites and occur in younger age groups
Keratoacanthoma	Rapidly growing nodule with horny central plug

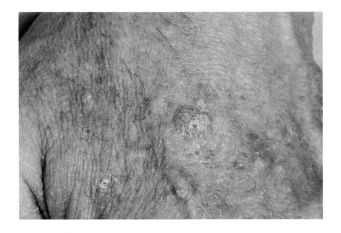

Figure 3.2

Multiple solar keratoses on the back of a man's hand.

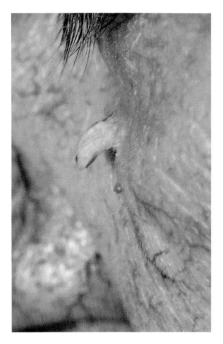

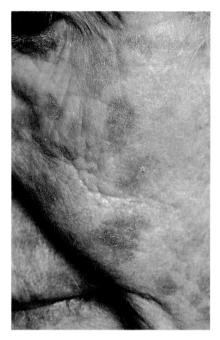

Figure 3.3

Cutaneous horn formed on a solar keratosis in a photodamaged man.

Figure 3.4

Multiple flat, red, slightly raised, scaling patches on the cheek of an elderly woman. These turned out to be solar keratoses although they could be mistaken for patches of discoid lupus erythematosus.

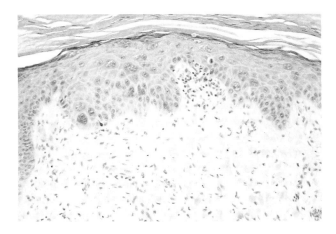

Figure 3.5

Histological section from lesion of solar keratosis showing cell heterogeneity and loss of polarity in an irregular epidermis.

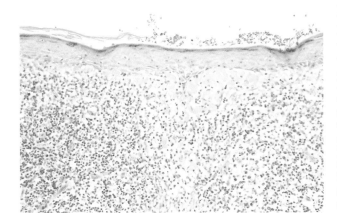

Figure 3.6

Histological section from a lesion on the face diagnosed as solar keratosis. There is considerable inflammation and erosion at the dermal–epidermal junction and numerous cytoid bodies characteristic of a lichenoid solar keratosis.

lesions there is also a marked subepidermal inflammatory cell infiltrate and even basal epidermal cell destruction, and a lichen planus-like appearance (Fig. 3.6). Abnormal mitotic figures and dyskeratotic cells within the epidermis are also observed. Bowen's disease is one stage further on (see Fig. 3.7) in the progression towards frank malignancy. The lesions tend to be plaque-like and scaling, especially on women's lower legs where they are not infrequently confused with plaques of psoriasis or of eczema (Fig. 3.8).

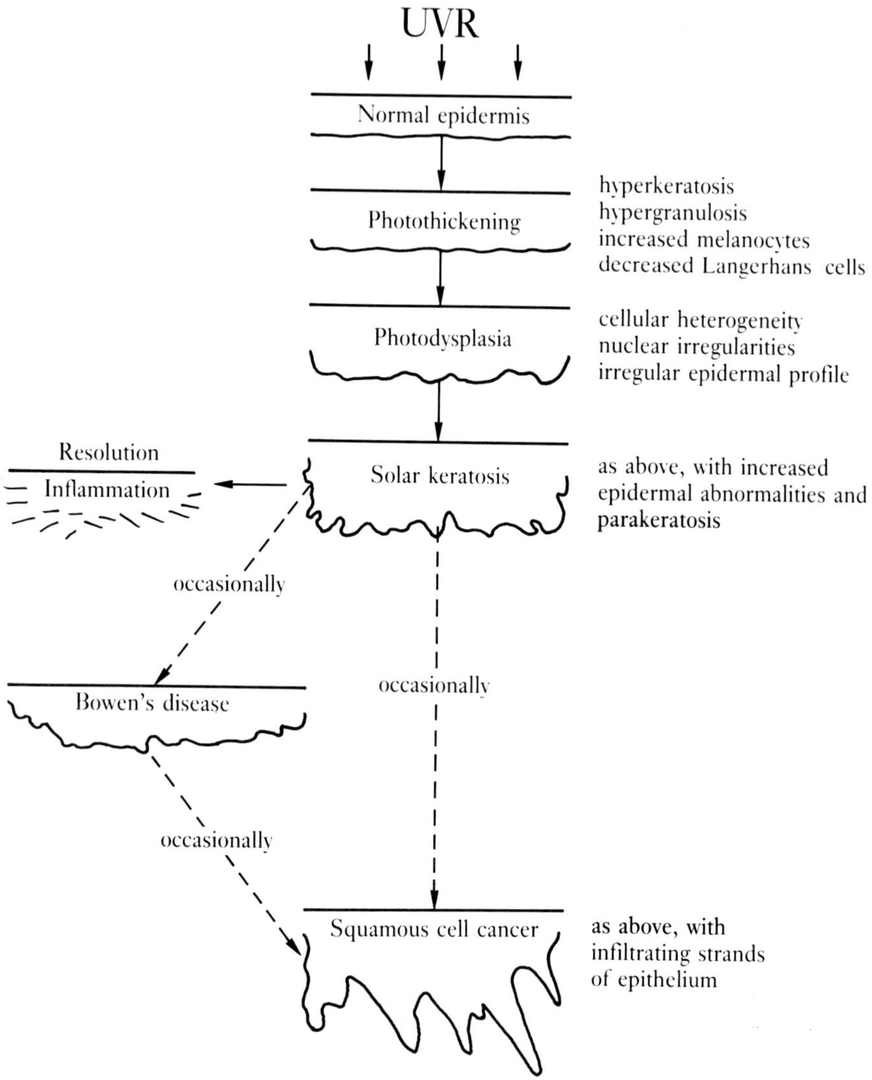

Figure 3.7

Sequence of events as a result of chronic
UVR damage to the epidermis.

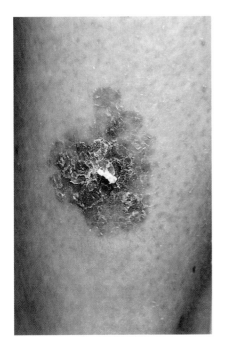

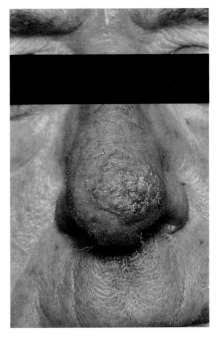

Figure 3.8

Plaque of Bowen's disease on the shin of a late middle-aged woman.

Figure 3.9

Plaque on the nose in an elderly man which turned out to be a squamous cell carcinoma.

Squamous cell carcinoma and keratoacanthoma

Further down the road there is frankly malignant squamous cell carcinoma. The question as to how frequently solar keratoses transform into these lesions has already been tackled (see page 37) but suffice to say here that it is very infrequent. Squamous cell carcinoma (SCC) is mainly but not exclusively the product of photodamage. It can also arise in areas damaged by heat and X-ray exposure in some unusual antigenic types of papilloma virus infection, and as a consequence of uncommon persistent inflammatory and destructive skin disorders such as lichen planus.

The condition should be suspected when a warty plaque enlarges and/or ulcerates (Figs 3.9 and 3.10). If the

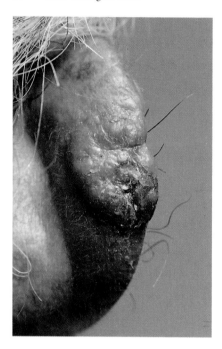

Figure 3.10

Eroded nodule on the ear caused by
squamous cell carcinoma.

lesion is highly aggressive, eroded
nodules develop (Fig. 3.11). Occasionally the epidermal tissue at the base
of a cutaneous horn may show histological characteristics of an SCC but
these lesions are slow-growing and
seem less infiltrative than other types.

It is often said that SCC of photodamaged skin metastasizes late, but as
it is sometimes difficult to distinguish
SCC histologically from the more

benign lesions of keratoacanthoma
(see below) and Bowen's disease, it is
difficult to accept this view totally. It is
not particularly uncommon to see
metastasizing lesions such as that
illustrated in Fig. 3.12 on the arm of a
60-year-old woman who subsequently
died from the disorder. However,
SCC lesions of mucosal surfaces (lips,
genitalia) do have a worse reputation.

Diagnosis is by biopsy, when
changes are observed that are quite
similar to but more pronounced than
those in solar keratosis. The epidermis
is markedly thickened with irregular
downgrowths into the epidermis (Fig.
3.13). At points vicarious differentiation is found which gives rise to 'horn
pearls' (Fig. 3.14). There is usually a
pronounced inflammatory cell infiltrate around the lesion.

Keratoacanthoma (KA) is the name
for an odd type of lesion that erupts
suddenly, takes on the characterstics
of an SCC and then subsides to
disappear—all within a period of 2–6
months. The typical KA has steep
sides and a central horny plug (Fig.
3.15). The problem in clinical diagnosis is that occasionally SCCs
look indistinguishable from KAs and
clearly the implications are quite different.

Unfortunately, histological differentiation is not always straightforward
either. There is a cup-shaped area
of epidermal hypertrophy projecting
into the dermis, the central cavity of
which contains horny debris. There is
a variable amount of inflammatory cell
infiltrate   and   one   characteristic

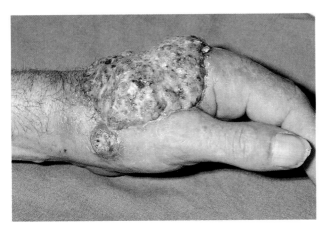

Figure 3.11

Massive eroded tumour on the back of the hand growing in size over the previous year in a welder who also showed considerable photo-damage.

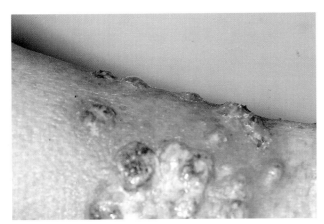

Figure 3.12

Metastasizing squamous cell carcinoma on the arm of a late middle-aged woman who showed considerable photodamage. This woman unfortunately died from her disease.

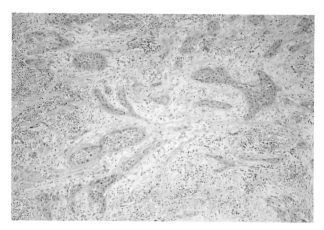

Figure 3.13

Histological section from squamous cell carcinoma showing infiltrating strands of abnormal epithelium in an inflamed fibrous stroma.

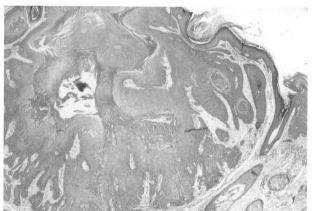

Figure 3.14

Histological section showing nodule of proliferation of epithelium due to squamous cell carcinoma.

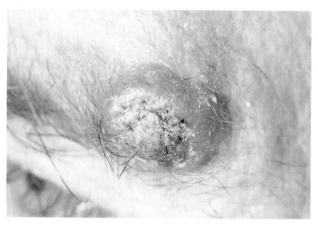

Figure 3.15

Typical keratoacanthoma with central horny plug.

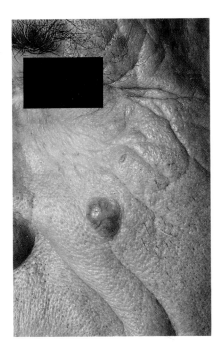

Figure 3.16

Pearly nodule typical of basal cell
carcinoma on the cheek of a
middle-aged man showing photodamage.

feature is the infiltration of the epidermal mass with polymorphs. Cellular and nuclear irregularity are not prominent but the presence of individual eosinophilic dyskeratotic cells is quite typical.

Basal cell carcinoma (BCC)

Basal cell carcinomas (BCCs) are common skin cancers known popularly as rodent ulcers, presumably because if left untreated they break down and the ulcerated plaque that remains has some kind of resemblance to a rat bite. Unlike squamous cell cancers there are no precursor lesions. As pointed out previously, although the large majority of these common lesions arise on sun-exposed skin, not all do. Some arise in developmental anomalies of the epidermis which include such conditions as naevus sebaceous and the basal cell naevus syndrome. The commonest clinical presentation of BCC is as an opalescent nodule or plaque over the nose, forehead or upper cheeks (Figs 3.16 and 3.17). Degenerative change in some lesions gives them a cystic appearance. The central parts of larger lesions break down to form an ulcer with a characteristic rolled margin (Fig. 3.18). There are several less common clinical variants of the basic cystic nodule plaque-type lesion. Occasionally lesions become darkly pigmented and may even be misdiagnosed as melanoma (Fig. 3.19). Less uncommon are superficial lesions whose growth potential seems to be directed horizontally rather than vertically. They appear as thin pink scaling plaques with fine, slightly raised and well-defined margins (Fig. 3.20). The least common and probably the most difficult to recognize is the morphoeic type. These resemble patches of localized scleroderma (morphoea) because of the accompanying fibrosis, and can be difficult to identify (Fig. 3.21). For the most part

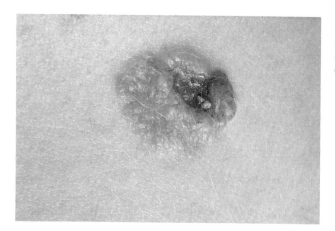

Figure 3.17

Eroded plaque
due to basal cell
carcinoma.

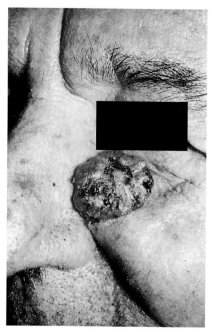

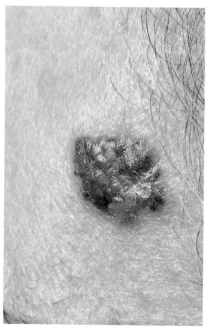

Figure 3.18

Large eroded nodule on the cheek,
caused by basal cell carcinoma.

Figure 3.19

Pigmented basal cell carcinoma.

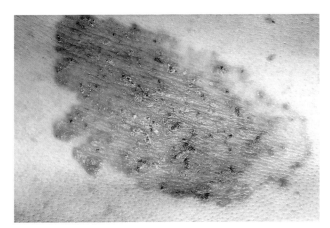

Figure 3.20

Superficial basal cell carcinoma. Note the well-defined, slightly raised edge.

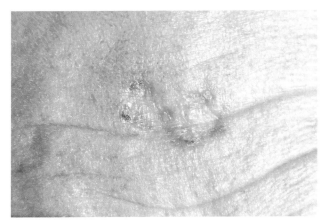

Figure 3.21

Depressed and infiltrated area on the forehead of a late middle-aged man which turned out to be a morphoeic basal cell carcinoma.

the BCC is locally invasive only and can be easily removed without a great deal of morbidity. Occasionally, however, the lesions are life-threatening because of extensive local infiltration or metastasis. The latter is rare, there being something of the order of 500 cases reported. Extensive local invasion with involvement of vital structures may be more of a problem especially around the eyes, ears and nose. The histological hallmark of BCC is the presence of clumps of basophilic cells in the dermis (Fig.

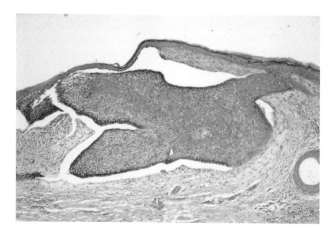

Figure 3.22

Histological section of a typical nodule of basal cell carcinoma.

3.22). The cells of the clumps show a surprising amount of mitotic activity as well as degenerative change. Around the clumps there is often a gap between the basaloid cells and the connective tissue. This is termed 're-traction artefact' and is due to the dissolving out of a colloid-like material from around the clumps. There is also a variable amount of fibrosis and inflammation.

Treatment of non-melanoma skin cancer and its precursors

A solitary solar keratosis or SCC or a BCC can be excised, subjected to curettage and cautery, or destroyed by cryotherapy or cautery. Only rarely is it necessary to resort to radiotherapy for the larger lesions or where the particular site or the age of the patient makes surgical treatment difficult. A 'cluster' of solar keratoses, a patch of Bowen's disease, or a superficial BCC can often be treated satisfactorily by an ointment containing 5% 5-fluorouracil daily for a 10-day period. The successfully treated patch often becomes quite sore before resolving. Care must be taken that too large an area is not treated in order to avoid systemic toxicity. Intra-lesional interferon-alpha 2β (1 million IU on each occasion, 3 times weekly for 3 weeks) has been used with considerable success to treat large solar keratoses, areas of Bowen's disease and BCCs. However, this treatment is expensive and inconvenient for the patient as well as causing systemic 'flu-like side-effects in some patients.

In addition to the above treatments, either systemic or topical retinoids may provide the appropriate help when patients have multiple lesions. Systemic etretinate or isotretinoin cause a reduction in the numbers of lesions as well as a reduction in their size while they are being given. This may be of considerable help for some patients who have large numbers of lesions in light-exposed sites, or who have multiple skin cancers on the basis of a genodermatosis such as xeroderma pigmentosum or the basal cell naevus syndrome. These drugs also have a prophylactic effect in that they appear to delay or inhibit the appearance of lesions in individuals who have an underlying predisposition to develop non-melanoma skin cancers.

Topical retinoids such as tretinoin have been used to treat multiple solar keratoses in large multicentre trials, and there can be little doubt that in severely photodamaged subjects with multiple lesions, there is a reduction in both the size and the number of visible lesions. As with systemic retinoids, the effects of topical tretinoin are mainly evident while the treatment is being used. It has also been suggested that topical tretinoin may be a useful treatment adjunct for use with 5% 5-fluorouracil when there are multiple solar keratoses.

Melanoma and Precursor Lesions

Because of the frightening rate of increase in the incidence of melanoma and precursor lesions, it is important that all who are likely to be consulted for small tumours of the skin—including dermatologists, surgeons and general practitioners—should learn how to differentiate melanoma from other pigmented lesions. Having said that, it must be admitted that even the most experienced dermatologist makes mistakes at times. Prospective studies suggest that with 'difficult to diagnose' lesions an accuracy rate of approximately 65–70% is all that can be expected even of experts.

Precursor lesions

Ordinary melanocytic naevi (moles) can certainly transform into melanomas but this in itself should not result in mass hypochondriasis. After all, the estimated lifetime risk for melanoma in the USA is less than 1%, and the incidence is perhaps six times less in Europe. Furthermore, one-half of melanomas arise from normal 'non-mole' skin. However, large congenital moles, that is, moles present from birth—and especially the so-called giant naevi of the 'cape' or 'bathing-trunk' type (Fig. 3.23)—have a much increased risk of developing melanoma. It has been suggested that 10%

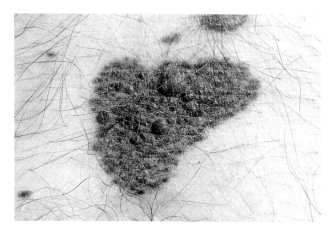

Figure 3.23

Large congenital type of mole. These seem more likely to transform into malignant melanoma than acquired naevi.

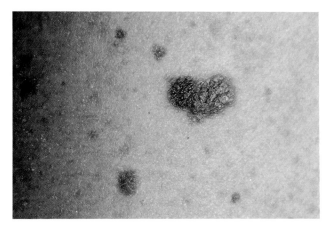

Figure 3.24

Example of an irregular and oddly coloured mole seen in the dysplastic naevus syndrome.

of such lesions develop a melanoma. The risk is also increased with larger numbers of moles.

'Dysplastic moles' are moles that have irregular features in that they are irregular in outline and variegate in colour (Figs 3.24 and 3.25). They also possess unusual and maybe disturbing histological features reminiscent of melanoma in some aspects. When many of these moles coexist in the same patient, the disorder is known as

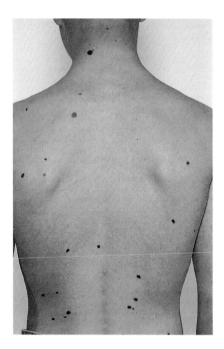

Figure 3.25

Young patient with many moles, some of which are oddly shaped and pigmented in a variegated fashion.

the dysplastic naevus syndrome. It is also known as the B.K. naevus syndrome after the initials of the patients who were first recognized as suffering from this problem.

The importance of this condition is the greatly increased risk of melanoma. It occurs sporadically but the condition is more often familial. It has been suggested that the risk of developing melanoma in an individual with the dysplastic mole syndrome is increased to 1% and that if a member of the family has had a melanoma previously, the risk is increased to 10%. Having developed one melanoma, there is a very high risk of developing another. Clearly it is important to recognize patients with this disorder, as they should be kept under surveillance. They need to be taught how to recognize the danger signals of transformation to a melanoma, and how to avoid solar radiation whenever possible. It is worth noting that some investigators do not accept that there is a separate disorder of the 'dysplastic mole syndrome', but do agree that there are patients with a greatly increased risk of melanoma.

Lentigo maligna (Hutchinson's freckle) is sometimes also known as melanoma *in situ*. Brown–black macules with 'festooned' or polycyclic margins varying in size from the quite small (0.5 cm^2) to the quite large (3 cm^2) are characteristic of the lesion (Fig. 3.26). The story often given by patients is that the area of pigmentation has gradually spread over a period of months or years. The temples, nose and cheeks are typical sites but the macules may also occur over the trunk. Lentigo maligna is not usually life-threatening unless a melanoma develops within the lesion, in which case the outlook is the same as for melanoma elsewhere. It is not uncommon for the pigmented macule to spread gradually over ten or more years without any serious effect.

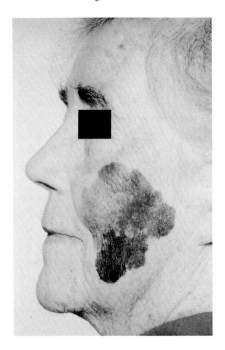

Figure 3.26

Lentigo maligna.

Melanoma

Danger signals

Change in the size, shape and colour of a mole and complaints of itching over a period of weeks or months suggest the development of melanoma (Table 3.2). Irregularity of the outline and surface, and variegation in colour are important physical signs (Fig. 3.27). Development of a pigmented

Table 3.2 Danger signs of melanoma

1   Increase in size of pre-existing mole or development of new pigmented lesion
2   Irregular outline developing in pre-existing mole or presence of this feature in new pigmented lesion
3   Irregular degree of pigmentation (variegation) in pre-existing mole or this feature in new pigmented lesion
4   Irritation, soreness, inflammation, crusting, erosion, bleeding in pre-existing mole or in new pigmented lesion

halo around the lesion is a late sign—as is the development of satellite nodules around the lesion. If left the melanoma will ulcerate but usually the diagnosis is established before this occurs.

It is important to confirm the diagnosis histologically before there are attempts at surgical ablation because, as mentioned previously, mistakes in the diagnosis of pigmented lesions are only too frequent. It is also important to note that the histological diagnosis is not always straightforward and is in the province of the expert dermatopathologist. For example, uncommon benign mole-like lesions are found in childhood which have many disturbing features histologically and, as with dysplastic naevi, it may be difficult to

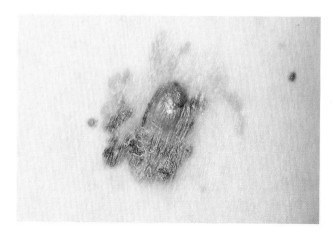

Figure 3.27

Nodule on varie-
gated plaque. This
turned out to be a
nodular malignant
melanoma.

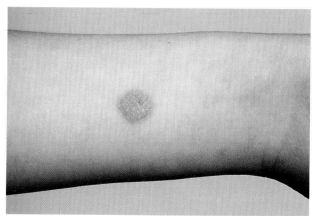

Figure 3.28

Red, plaque-like
lesion on the arm
of a child, typical
of juvenile melan-
oma.

distinguish them from malignant melanoma. These lesions are called juvenile melanomas but they are quite harmless and need not be removed if recognized as such, by the fact that they are found in children and have a pinkish-red–orange surface (Fig. 3.28).

Melanoma is a potentially fatal lesion. If left until it has metastasized treatment is difficult and inadequate and most patients are dead within two years. The prognosis depends entirely on the depth of invasion within the skin. The so-called 'nodular' melanoma (Fig. 3.29) tends to spread

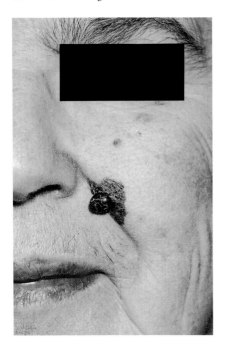

Figure 3.29
Nodular melanoma of the cheek.

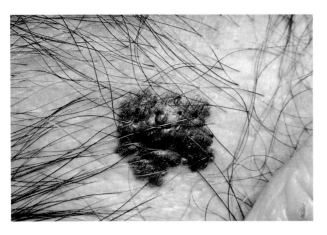

Figure 3.30
Superficial spreading melanoma on the chest of a middle-aged man.

downwards and has a poor prognosis, whilst the 'superficial' melanoma (Fig. 3.30) tends to spread horizontally and has a much better outlook. If the melanoma reaches the deep part of the dermis or more than 1.7 mm the 5-year survival rate is less than 80%. If the lesion has not penetrated to more than 0.7 mm then there is a good chance of cure and a five-year survival rate of more than 95%.

Treatment of melanoma

The treatment of melanoma is essentially surgical. Most dermatologists agree that if there is any suspicion of there being a melanoma, the lesion in question should be removed with a 3-mm margin as soon as possible. If the diagnosis is confirmed histologically, then most suggest that the excision site is re-excised soon after.

Major primary excisions and lymph-node clearance are now not often performed unless there are specific indications from knowledge of the spread of the disease.

Lentigo maligna is sometimes treated by radiotherapy but in general melanoma tissue is not very radiosensitive. Lentigo maligna has also been treated by cryotherapy but this is not recommended as the fall in tissue temperature is not sufficient deeper in the dermis where some of the abnormal cells may reach.

When melanoma has spread, several types of treatment have been used including chemotherapeutic agents such as melphalan, retinoids and interferons. In general, these have at best provided only temporary and partial remissions and there is a desparate need for new and more effective agents.

4

Protection from the Sun

The most effective way of avoiding sun damage is to avoid the sun but few people are likely to take any note of this counsel of perfection. Currently, most of the population seem to want to be outdoors and in the sun whenever possible and it is important to give advice on how to avoid serious UVR exposure when individuals are involved in outdoor activities.

Simple measures are best. If there is adequate shade then it should be used. Dappled shade is not adequate. Even in comparatively 'solid' shade there is some solar UVR that reaches exposed skin and this will depend on the nature of the objects giving the shade and on the distance away from surfaces receiving direct sun. It will also depend on the nature of the terrain. White surfaces reflect back considerable amounts of UVR, increasing the amount of UVR that can reach the skin directly. Snow is particularly efficient at reflecting UVR; expanses of water and sandy beaches are less efficient but are nonetheless reflecting surfaces. Clearly, individuals should be warned as to the increased risk of

significant solar damage when skiing and sailing. Incidentally, it is easy to be fooled when swimming. The cool sensation of being in the water does not prevent sunburn: even swimming in deep water does not protect, as UVR penetrates water easily. Skiing is a particular problem where, because of the increased altitude, there is less filtration out of the UVR by the atmosphere and consequently increased opportunity for high doses of UVR to reach the skin.

The worst time of the day as far as solar UVR exposure is concerned is around midday, and it is prudent to emphasize that if individuals insist on exposing themselves, they should try to avoid the hours 11a.m.–2p.m. Obviously summer is the time for particular caution and in the Western hemisphere June–September are the danger months. This is not to say that it is impossible to be injured by solar UVR outside these times. It is possible to be badly damaged by the sun in February–May in subtropical areas (as once happened to the author in Miami in February). Even in temperate climates sunburn is possible in May or October if the individual remains in the direct sun for some time.

One further point that is worth bearing in mind concerns the possibility of solar damage when the sky is overcast. Cloud cover may not give much protection from the sun especially when the cloud is thin and wispy.

A certain amount of sun protection can be obtained from clothing. Broad-brimmed hats (Stetsons, Canadian Mounties' hats and ladies' Ascot-type creations are ideal) provide considerable protection for the face. Certainly, some kind of headgear is *de rigueur* for bald-headed individuals such as the author. Thin blouses and skirts do not offer much protection and it is not uncommon to find that sunburn occurs on the back and chest of people wearing such garments.

Sunscreen Preparations

Sunscreens are important adjuncts for skin protection and will be needed to supplement any advice given. There are a vast number of such preparations and in recent years they have become a major part of the cosmetics–toiletries market. Essentially, there are two main varieties of sunscreen—preparations that reflect the sun's rays and preparations that filter out the harmful UVR. Historically, the first preparation to be used extensively was distributed to soldiers in the Second World War and was known as 'Red Vet Pet'. This substance was made of an iron oxide suspended in petroleum jelly. It was thick, greasy, gave a bizarre appearance and to all accounts was unpleasant to use. However, it gave excellent protection against sunburn! Red Vet Pet reflected away all incident solar UVR and not an inconsiderable amount of the visible light as well, in addition to giving some protection against infrared radiation.

Similar protection on the basis of reflectance can also be obtained by the use of preparations containing zinc oxide and titanium dioxide. The latter in particular has been employed in sunscreens. The major problem with these types of product is that it is difficult to make them cosmetically acceptable. Their ability to reflect solar UVR also gives them the property of reflecting visible light so that after application to the skin patients look like circus clowns. Recently it has been possible to make titanium dioxide of a very fine particle size so that it is possible for the preparation to reflect predominantly UVR rather than visible wavelengths. This type of sunscreen has a major advantage in that it reflects both UVA and UVB (see later).

Sun protection factor

A moment's thought will indicate why it is useful to have a system which makes it possible to categorize the efficiency of sunscreen products. Subjects who are very sensitive to the sun need the most protective preparations. Exposure to sunlight of high intensity demands a highly protective sunscreen regardless of sensitivity.

A sunscreen's protective capacity is expressed for UVB and UVA (see Chapter 1) separately because there are no materials that give protection equally across the UVR spectrum. In the case of UVB the sun protection factor (SPF) is the time required to produce the minimal degree of erythema when using the preparation (T_p) divided by the time required to produce the minimal degree of erythema without any protection (T), i.e. SPF = T_p/T. This sounds easier than it is in practice. Rigorous standardization is required to ensure that the SPF is a reproducible value regardless of the laboratory in which the determination is made. The standardization is currently imposed by governmental agencies in the USA, Australia and Germany. Unfortunately, the details of the way the SPF tests are made differ between the above three agencies so that a cream tested in Germany using the recommended method and found to have an SPF of 10 may have a different SPF when tested according to Australian guidelines. The major difference relates to the artificial source of UVR with which the tests are made. The German protocol, which is currently under review, requires a lamp that emits at particular wavelengths, whilst the USA and Australian agencies demand that the UVR source is a solar simulator, that is, a lamp that emits a continuous spectrum. The tests are run with panels of volunteer subjects and another difference relates to the number of individuals in the panel tested. Other differences are concerned with the amount of sunscreen put on the skin surface and the way that the lamps are shone on the skin.

This type of SPF testing is important but suitable only for testing products that protect against UVB. This is because UVA does not produce erythema very easily and other endpoints need to be chosen if the tests are to be made in human volunteers. A variety of test systems have been devised to test for protection against UVA, including 'immediate pigment darkening' in which the skin is examined for darkening very shortly after irradiation, and protection against psoralens and photosensitization. A much better method is to employ an *in vitro* technique in which the sunscreen is applied to a transparent membrane of some kind and the transmission of UVR through the membrane with and without the material is determined using a radiometer device. The SPF for UVA is then (transmission of UVA with material) divided by (transmission of UVA without material).

Inspection of the tubes and packages of sunscreen preparations in the high street will reveal that very few carry much information about their UVA protection. This is because it is only relatively recently that it has been recognized that UVA is a potential source of skin damage. This could be a quite serious problem for individuals who use an efficient UVB protecting sunscreen—it would stop them being sunburnt but would allow long-term damage to accumulate from UVA! The other major reasons for there being little information about UVA protection are that there are few safe and efficient substances that adequately protect against UVA that are suitable for use in sunscreens, and that, as pointed out above, it is difficult to test them.

There are many materials used in sunscreens and the most popular of these are set out in Table 4.1. For the most part these preparations are very safe to use but it should be noted that the fact that chemicals absorb certain wavelengths means that they are 'photoactivated' and if absorbed into the skin some can cause a dermatitis. However, this should not deter from recommending their use on every conceivable occasion. Amongst the best sunscreens are those that contain titanium dioxide since, apart from protecting against UVB, they also provide substantial protection against UVA. However, unless titanium di-

oxide sunscreens are applied as a very thin even film, they produce a white 'ghostly' appearance to the user.

Apart from absorbing harmful radiation, sunscreens should have other qualities. In particular, they should adhere well to the skin surface and resist being easily washed off, both important properties if they are going to be used—as most of them are—on the beach. It is also vital that sunscreen preparations are pleasant to use and do not feel tacky or greasy. If they are not cosmetically acceptable they will not be used; and they will not prevent much skin cancer if they stay in the bottle!

In general it is advisable that a sunscreen protects adequately against both UVB and UVA. For the most part

Table 4.1 Examples of substance used in sunscreens

Group	Specific example	Type	Protects against
Esters of para-aminobenzoic acid	Padimate	Filter	UVB
Esters of cinnamic acid	Ethylhexyl *p*-methoxy-cinnamate	Filter	UVB + some UVA
Benzophenones	Oxybenzone	Filter	UVB + some UVA
Titanium dioxide	Micronized titanium	Reflectant	UVB and UVA
Salicylates	Homomenthyl salicylates	Filter	UVB
Anthranilates	Menthyl anthranilate	Filter	UVA

sunscreens with SPFs for UVB in the region of 12–14 are suitable for use by most people in Europe (except perhaps very sensitive Type I and II subjects in the sunniest parts of the Mediterranean and Adriatic). Very sensitive people—particularly the red-haired and those who freckle easily—should use even higher SPF preparations in the region of 18–20, especially if skiing, yachting, surfing or mountaineering. There is not much purpose to preparations with SPFs in excess of 20. Unfortunately it is difficult to give much advice with regard to UVA protection other than to ensure that the preparation does possess protective properties in this region of the spectrum and that they very approximately match the UVB protection offered. It is useful to remember that the level of UVA reaching the Earth's surface is very similar in both summer and winter.

Orally Protective Agents

There are no drugs which when taken by mouth completely protect against solar UVR. However, there are some agents that partly protect. The best known and most used is beta-carotene. This is the orange–yellow precursor of vitamin A but when large amounts are taken it is deposited in the epidermis and stratum corneum, imparting a characteristic colour to the skin that is most noticeable on the palms and soles. It has been found that this drug does protect against wavelengths right on the border between UVA and blue light, which is important in preventing lesions in the disorder of porphyrin metabolism known as erythropoietic protoporphyria. Canthexanthin is another, not dissimilar compound—an analogue of beta-carotene. It has been used especially for the golden colour it gives the skin—a sort of pseudo-sunburn. This material was on sale over the counter but has been withdrawn because crystals of the substance were found deposited in the retina and there have been doubts as to its safety. The antimalarials—particularly mepacrine—give some protection against the sun but they are now rarely used for this purpose.

5

Treatments for Photodamage

There is a strong probability that if further photodamage is prevented then repair takes place in both the dermis and the epidermis. However, there is no evidence to support this hypothesis, mainly because it is extremely difficult to organize and complete long-term studies that could answer this question. In any event, it has to be sensible advice to avoid further sun damage whatever other treatment modality is advised.

Drug Treatments

Treatments for solar keratoses and various sun-induced skin cancers were partly dealt with in Chapter 3.

Topical retinoic acid

Over the past 6–7 years the news that topical all-*trans*-retinoic acid (tretinoin, Retin-A) can produce consider-able improvement in the clinical signs of photodamage has bemused and excited both the medical and the lay press. This has provoked a fascinating debate at several levels. One aspect of the discussion has been whether solar damage is a 'disease' that merits drug treatment, or whether it is an unfortunate concomitant of the passing of the years and is more in the province of the cosmetician than the doctor. As will be evident from previous chapters, the author's view is that photodamage represents a preventable, environmentally induced disease in which there is compromised structure and function of skin, and a tendency to develop skin cancer. It is reasonable to draw comparisons with the admittedly more life-threatening disorders due to alcoholism and tobacco addiction. Few would doubt that the results of these habits merit formal medical treatment. Why then should there be a distinction between these conditions and those produced by injudicious exposure to the sun? Whether the treatments for photodamage should be a cost to government-funded health services or not is another issue and one which goes far beyond the boundaries set for this book.

The medical debate has also been of great interest. There can be little doubt from the carefully conducted clinical trials conducted so far, that tretinoin improves the objective signs of photodamage. The point at issue has been whether the action is specific or whether it is based on the irritant and oedema-inducing properties of

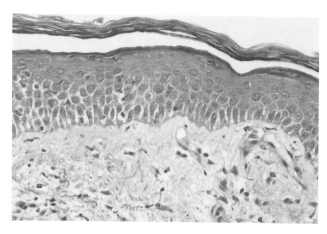

Figure 5.1

Section from area of normal skin treated with 1% dithranol showing an irritant reaction with spongiosis and epidermal thickening.

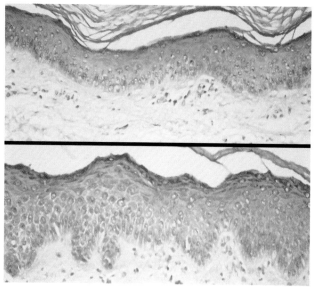

Figure 5.2

Two histological sections taken from an area treated by a bland emollient cream (upper) and an area treated with tretinoin 0.05% for 3 months (lower). There is epidermal thicken-ing, some increase in thickness of the granular layer and a change in the appearance of the stratum corneum – all typical of tretinoin-treated skin.

the drug. The histological evidence seems to rule out there being an inflammatory response in the skin such as is seen with alkalis or detergents (Fig. 5.1). There are few inflammatory cells and little oedema observed in tretinoin-treated skin. The prominent alteration is seen in the epidermis, which thickens quite markedly (Fig. 5.2). In addition, the stratum corneum also becomes compacted and looks quite different from

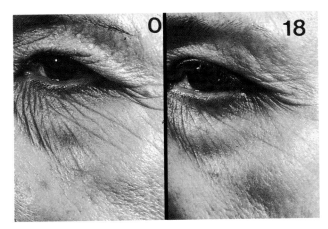

Figure 5.3
Treatment with
0.1% tretoinin.
(a) Before and
after 18 months'
treatment.
(b) Before and
after 20 months'
treatment.
(Reproduced with
kind permission
from Dr John
Voorhees.)

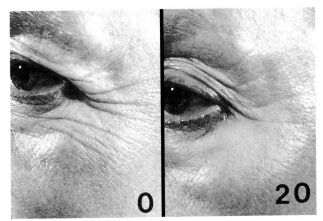

the profile in untreated skin. It has also been reported that more blood vessels and new dermal connective tissue occurring immediately below the epidermis develop in tretinoin-treated skin. It must be said that these structural alterations have been described only rarely and then only in the skin of subjects treated with topical tretinoin for several years. They have also been demonstrated in animal models. They have not been found, as yet, in the course of formal controlled clinical trials.

Do these histological changes signify that tretinoin exerts its effects in photodamaged skin via specific and retinoid receptor-linked pathways? There is at present no definitive answer to this question. It seems likely that a proportion of the effects are retinoid-specific but that a significant proportion are not. It is certainly the case that some of the alterations recorded in the skin can be mimicked by the use of an abrasive preparation. Clearly, tissue repair mechanisms are initiated by topical tretinoin whatever the details of the cellular apparatus involved.

At the time of writing it is uncertain just how much photodamage is capable of repair. The published photographs (e.g. Fig. 5.3) certainly suggest that a quite remarkable improvement can occur in both the fine lines and in the deeper wrinkles at the sides of the eyes and mouth. In addition, skin colour improves and solar lentigines gradually decrease in prominence. As mentioned in Chapter 3, treatment with topical tretinoin also reduces the number of solar keratoses present.

The effects appear to be dose-related in that the most dramatic effects are observed with 0.1% tretinoin and less marked changes occur with the 0.05% and 0.025% concentrations. Proponents of tretinoin preparations for photodamage suggest that it should be rubbed into the face at night and that a sunscreen should be used during the day.

Tretinoin side-effects

Preparations of tretinoin tend to make the skin feel sore and slightly rougher than usual but these side-effects are usually mild and tolerable and anyway tend to decrease with time. Some patients complain that they are more sensitive to the sun when using topical tretinoin and they should be warned of this possibility. This sensitivity probably results from the stratum corneum being thinner on account of the increased rate of desquamation with the drug.

All retinoid drugs are teratogenic and the possible risks to the unborn child from the use of topical tretinoin during pregnancy have been researched quite extensively. Very little tretinoin is actually absorbed through the skin—not more than 2% in most studies. It should be noted that tretinoin is a natural metabolite of vitamin A and that no increases can be found in the normal blood level of this compound after experimental application to the skin. Furthermore, no reports of fetal malformation resulting from the use of topical tretoinoin have appeared despite the product being available for the treatment of acne since 1971.

The question of the carcinogenicity of topical tretinoin has also been investigated extensively. At the time of writing the position is that although in some experiments in mice there appears to be increased tumour formation from UVR, in others there is no such increase and there is no indication that topical tretinoin acts as a photocarcinogen in man.

Other retinoids

Topical isotretinoin has also been used in clinical trials for photodamage. Interestingly, the results indicate a marked decrease in the signs of solar elastosis after use for some months. There are other topical retinoids that have been reported to be helpful in photodamage but the published results are too scant to comment further. The most important conclusion to be drawn from studies with isotretinoin and other retinoids is that a therapeutic effect in chronic photodamage is not confined to tretinoin.

Other topical agents

As most readers will realize, claims for improvement in wrinkling have been made for a vast array of products ranging from extracts of various animals' organs and fetal tissues to vitamin E. Little scientific evidence exists to support these claims. Interesting work has been reported with elastin-containing products, but more data are required before any conclusions can be drawn.

The Surgical Approach to Photodamage

Prior to the use of topical retinoids the only treatment possible for photodamage was cosmetic surgery. Indeed, cosmetic surgical manoeuvres are still employed for many subjects who are severely affected who require a 'quick fix' and who can afford the cost. Facial 'tightening' procedures to smooth out wrinkles, and 'tucks', if performed by experienced surgeons, can produce considerable improvement in appearance, especially for lines at the sides of the eyes and sagging skin of the neck. The detail of the various manoeuvres adopted is beyond the scope of this work and the interested reader is advised to consult one of the many skin surgery texts available.

Chemical peeling with phenol or trichloroacetic acid produces a superficial burn on the skin, and when performed by experienced dermatologists is seen to produce some improvement in the clinical appearance. The same can be said of intradermal collagen injections. These fill in the hollows and can help to smooth out lines and furrows. These improvements are, however, temporary, and treatment needs to be repeated at regular intervals.

Further Reading

Balin AK, Kligman AM, eds (1989). *Aging and the Skin*. New York: Raven Press.

Dalziel K (1991). Aspects of cutaneous ageing. *Clinical & Experimental Dermatology* 16: 315–323.

Epstein JH (1983). Photocarcinogenesis, skin cancer, and aging. *Journal of the American Academy of Dermatology* 9: 487–502.

Harvey I, Frankel SJ, Shalom SD, and Marks R (1989). Non melanoma skin cancer: Questions concerning its distribution and natural history. *British Medical Journal* 299: 1118–1120.

Kligman AM, Grove GL, Hirose R et al. (1986). Topical tretinoin for photoaged skin. *Journal of the American Academy of Dermatology* 15: 836–859.

Marks R (1986). Premalignant disease of the epidermis (Parkes Weber Lecture 1985). *Journal of the Royal College of Physicians of London* 20: 116–121.

Marks R, ed. (1991). *Retinoids in Cutaneous Malignancy*. Oxford: Blackwell Scientific Publications.

Index

Page numbers in *italic* refer to the illustrations